EATING CLEAN

DETOX, REDUCE WEIGHT, FIGHT INFLAMMATION AND RESET YOUR BODY

BY SMART READS

Free Audiobook

As a thank you for being a Smart Reader you can choose 2 FREE audiobooks from audible.com. Simply sign up for free by visiting www.audibletrial.com/Travis to get your books.

Visit:
www.smartreads.co/freebooks
to receive Smart Reads books for FREE

Check us out on Instagram:
www.instagram.com/smart_readers
@smart_readers

ABOUT SMARTREADS

Choose Smart Reads and get smart every time. Smart Reads sorts through all the best content and condenses the most helpful information into easily digestible chunks.

We design our books to be short, easy to read and highly informative. Leaving you with maximum understanding in the least amount of time.

Smart Reads aims to accelerate the spread of quality information so we've taken the copyright off everything we publish and donate our material directly to the public domain. You can read our uncopyright below.

We believe in paying it forward and donate 5% of our net sales to **Pencils of Promise** to build schools, train teachers and support child education.

To limit our footprint and restore forests around the globe we are planting a tree for every 10 hardcover books we sell.

Thanks for choosing Smart Reads and helping us help the planet.

Sincerely,

Travis & the Smart Reads Team

TABLE OF CONTENTS

INTRODUCTION

Life today is more stressful than ever that's why staying healthy in mind and body is essential. Within these pages you will find information to guide you in the right direction to achieving a healthy lifestyle.

The first thing that must be done is to honestly analyze your own eating habits. Many of us will choose to eat things like coffee and donuts in the morning, or perhaps some type of cereal, which can be loaded with sugar. At lunchtime or in the evening our meals are not much better. Due to the usual office routines, many people have little time for preparing or having proper meals and opt for fast food and not necessarily nutritious. Burgers, pizza, and lasagna are amongst the most popular foods for this time of the day. Often at dinnertime, restaurants are full of people asking for "junk" food.

If we stop and think carefully about the food we eat on a daily basis we'll find so much of it is artificially processed. Very little of the food we eat is whole food or natural food. Artificially processed foods are full of artificial flavors and even chemicals. This being the case, you can then begin to imagine that it wouldn't be very healthy for the body. How then, can we stay healthy and disease free when the food we put in our bodies is unnatural?

The good news is that it's not too late and we can change our eating habits. We can begin to live a new and healthy life by making a few small changes.

Changing our diet and eating healthy is not about choosing food in pretty packaging and allowing this to fool us into thinking it is nutritious. Eating healthy means choosing whole food items that contain natural flavors and content; food that lets us know what we're getting. Healthy eating means adding things like fruit and vegetables to our eating habits. These are some of the whole foods mentioned before. They are foods whereby we can see exactly what we're getting because the food is whole, not chopped up and mixed with a lot of other things that we don't even know what they are.

Other whole foods include seafood, meats, and whole cereals. These, along with fruit and vegetables, all play an essential role in keeping our bodies healthy and providing the right amount of fiber, vitamins and minerals. Seafood and meat help the body build protein levels naturally and will not make us addicted to things such as artificially processed protein packs which are readily available to us in the marketplace.

This book will provide you with clear explanations and details of how to eat clean and provide easy recipes you can make yourself for breakfast, for lunch and for dinner; recipes that will boost the immune system to make you stronger and maintain good health for the long term.

Don't go to the gym and bring with you preservative drinks or food to eat afterwards. Stick to natural foods. Allow your stamina to build naturally. Research has shown that people who eat simply and have a fresh diet tend to live longer and healthier lives. Those who stick to a lot of processed food and "junk food" which are usually artificially processed tend to have more health problems earlier in life. This type of food will damage the stomach lining, as well as the liver and the kidneys in the long run due to the high number of unnatural chemicals used in it.

The recipes contained in this book have been chosen because of their nutritional value and the fact that they have very few, if any, artificial additives or chemicals.
Combination food recipes such as omelets, smoothies, milkshakes, gravies, and also desserts, will provide you with nutrition and variety.

CHAPTER 1: CLEAN EATING BASICS

In today's world, with all the hustle and bustle and the lack of time, clean eating habits have taken a back seat with many people. We have begun to rely so much on the ready-made, easy-to-grab food items to satisfy our taste buds. This is producing both minor health issues and major ones. Issues such as leaky gut syndrome, cholesterol problems, obesity, and an immune system failure have become all too common and prevalent. So many health campaigns and seminars are being promoted these days by health professionals and sometimes by the government itself to educate people about the benefits of healthy eating.

Eating out is something so many of us do on a regular basis. There is nothing wrong with this per se, and of course, we should have the option to go out. However, not all food places maintain high hygiene levels that the body needs. Sometimes, people begin to feel ill without knowing why.

Clean Eating – What Is It?
When we use the words "clean eating" it does not refer to the state of the cutlery or crockery, even though of course, they must be clean too. Rather, clean eating refers to the food we are eating - that it must contain clean properties. Clean food is good organic

food that hasn't been tampered with preservatives, flavorings and other chemicals. It refers to things like fresh fruit and vegetables, naturally processed dairy, seafood, lean meat and also whole grains. Other things such as healthy oils are also essential to maintain a good diet.

If you want to change your eating habits then this book and its information is for you. Changing your old eating practices and starting new healthier ones can be done easily. Don't wait any longer. Start with boosting your immune system. Let's begin the journey together now.

Limit Processed Food Consumption

So much of what we eat today is actually artificial. Canned foods, sweets, chocolates, processed dairy, artificially processed meats etc., have become the new "natural." Processed foods are composed of so many chemicals and these are harming our bodies in major ways. These chemicals have the potential to hurt our immune systems and our endocrine systems. In turn, once our endocrine system is compromised we suffer problems with hormone control – affecting how our body functions including our mood and even mental state. Mood swings and depression have become normal among average people.

Take chicken, for example. In many cases they are genetically grown and fed certain chemically laden food to make them grow faster and bigger. This is not healthy and the chicken meat lacks basic nutritional protein. Some scientists claim this type of chicken is machine meat, destructive to our health and tasteless.

Avoiding as much processed and artificial food as you can is a good start if you decide to change to healthier eating. Look for farm chickens or farm meat; choose fresh fruit and vegetables instead of canned or packed goods, which have been sitting, in a freezer for long periods of time.

Be Aware of Your Sodium Intake
Appropriate amounts of sodium are necessary to maintaining a healthy and appropriate mineral composition within the body. Most Americans will eat lower levels of sodium they need, and African Americans tend to take more sodium than necessary. This leads to higher blood pressure, diabetes, and kidney disease.

Be aware and careful of the amount of sodium you are putting in your body. Avoid ready-made marinating sauces for meats for example, as they contain very high sodium levels and they are not good for your health. You could do more of the cooking yourself at home where you can be sure of the hygiene levels. When you start cooking from the start, you have full control over how much of any ingredient and what types of ingredients go into your food.

Consume Less Meat

Even though meat helps our health in terms of being a main protein source, iron, and vitamin B12, you must choose meat that has not been artificially processed. Eating too much of anything is not good and this goes for meat. Meat takes more time to digest and for some people leaves a very heavy feeling in the body. Eating too much meat or the wrong type can also lead to having high cholesterol and blood pressure, even heart problems. Try eating smaller portions of meat cooked in healthy oils and add more vegetables to your meals.

Vegetables Are Best

Fresh vegetables are our best friends. Nothing is better than eating fresh vegetables. They contain so much fiber, vitamins and minerals. Eating a proper amount of fresh, nutritious vegetables have helped people cure and deal with certain illnesses. Vegetables are versatile and can be cooked and consumed in different ways, including eating them raw. Every vegetable contains its own important benefits for the body. They are best-consumed fresh and when they are in season.

Choose Whole Grains

Our bodies need whole grains and therefore we must take them in adequate amounts. The most popular are rice dishes and of course, are always more hygienic when made at home complemented with some meat or vegetables. Whole wheat has benefits so choose whole grains whenever you can.

Eating clean does not only benefit oneself but also the entire family. Cooking and eating clean, healthy, nutritious food will ensure all family members are eating well and staying healthier. Using the guidelines available in this book will help you cook well and eat well.

CHAPTER 2: GETTING STARTED

Now that you are better informed about what clean food and clean eating is and isn't, we will begin to put a daily routine into practice.

We must begin to train our minds first because after many years of doing one thing it will take a little while to switch to another. Be kind to yourself while this process is occurring. Keep reminding yourself that from this moment on you will do what you must in order to get yourself and your family healthier and stronger.

Sometimes, people start their new eating habits with gusto but let the enthusiasm dwindle out after a little while due to old habits that were formed in childhood. You will need to be consistent so you'll have to train your mind and then begin the transformation process.

Adhere to the Clean Eating Rules
Following a clean eating pattern is like anything else in life. We must create the right mindset and work on ourselves. Look at the ideas below to help you start changing your habits.

- Avoid White: skip the sugar and the white flour because it usually has drastic effects on our bodies. Anything white is artificially processed and contains many artificial chemicals. Sugar is like a slow motion poison and causes an addiction in the body. It destroys it eventually. Diabetes has become an epidemic in today's modern world.

- Avoid Alcohol: Alcohol destroys nearly every organ in the body and can be dangerous especially in high amounts. Never add wine to the food you are cooking. It destroys the freshness and often contaminates it.
- Choose Healthy Fats: Not all fats are bad. Some of them are good and necessary for the body. Make sure you use the healthy ones such as olive oil, coconut oil and other nut oils. There is a reason the Mediterranean diet has been researched extensively. Start cooking your food using olive oil, which is very healthy.
- Consume Fresh Everything: Choose fresh fruit, vegetables, and farm meat. On your shopping trip always choose fresh fruit and vegetables, avoid canned or packed goods. Fresh food contains more vitamins, minerals, and fiber. A diet that is healthy will contain a combination of lean meat,

vegetables and fruit for lunch and also for dinner.

Clean Out The Fridge

Make sure you have a fridge that will be able to hold all the fresh edibles you will be bringing home. A fridge needs to be clean space-wise, but also physically clean so that bacteria and fungus won't thrive. Clean out your fridge and put your new, healthy food in it.

Allow Yourself a Treat Sometimes

Of course, sticking consistently to a new way of eating can be challenging. However, there's no need to deny yourself treats all the time. Choose a day and allow yourself to eat what you want without feeling guilty about it. Just be sure to make this day perhaps once a week and not every other day. Saturday or Sunday are the most popular days for treating oneself, probably because a lot of people will go out or have special plans on these days. Too much restriction will feel like you are punishing yourself.

Clean the Kitchen Benches and Cabinets

Make sure your kitchen in general is clean. You will be preparing food and using bench tops, cabinets etc. Make sure the entire area is clean. Wipe down everything to remove bacteria. If your kitchen isn't clean enough sometimes bacteria or germs from surrounding areas might rest on the food you have taken out and cause health problems.

Prepare a Grocery List

Once you have made the decision to change old eating habits you will also have to change the way you shop. You will have to be better prepared and plan ahead instead of just picking up the easiest thing you can find in the supermarket. Before you leave home, make a grocery list and include the items you must buy: fresh fruit and vegetables, farm fresh meat or poultry, or naturally processed dairy. Don't buy these things in bulk as they will lose their freshness and nutritional value if they sit in the fridge too long and. Meat can be frozen and kept for around 3 months before defrosting. Make sure you never defrost a piece of meat and then freeze it again. This will cause bacteria to grow and cause gastric problems.

Schedule Cooking Time

We are all so busy with kids, jobs, and other engagements and therefore it is important for us to make sure we have the time to cook for our families and ourselves. Schedule a time when you can prepare what you need in advance. If you would like to make some pickled vegetables or jams, for example, you will have to make time during the weekend perhaps, to make them and then stock them. This way you have them ready and handy whenever you need them, at least for the next few weeks.

Make a Menu Schedule

It's a good idea to have a menu schedule. This could be something you put on the fridge so you can look at it and get the things you need before the meal day arrives. A scheduling menu will save you time from having to figure out what you will cook every day. It will also help you balance what you will eat to ensure you get the vitamins, minerals and fiber you need from day to day. After a little while you will become accustomed to the schedule and probably won't need to look at it so much. The routine will be in your head.

CHAPTER 3: BREAKFAST

Breakfast is important as it gives us the kick-start we need for the day. It also helps to maintain energy levels throughout the day. Below are some really good recipes you can follow. They will help you avoid artificial type food as you focus more on natural ones that are good for your health.

Recipe 1: Mixed Berry Smoothie

Ingredients: (serves one)
½ Cup almond, coconut milk, (or hemp seed)
½ Cup of frozen or fresh strawberries
½ cup of frozen or fresh blueberries
½ Cup of blackberries
1 or 2 dates

Process: Place all the above ingredients into a clean blender. Blend them together to make a smoothie. This is all-natural and doesn't contain any chemicals or preservatives, so it can be added to your healthy, clean eating schedule. It contains lots of fiber and immune boosting fruits too.

Recipe 2: Coconut Water and Banana Smoothie

Combining both coconut water and banana will provide you with a healthy mix of ingredients. This particular recipe also includes avocado as well as hemp seeds. These are main sources of protein and provide great benefits to your diet overall.

In this recipe, we have included wheatgrass and cacao nibs, both of which play an essential role in providing magnesium to our bodies. Magnesium is an important element that helps maintain energy levels, in particular with athletes. If you regularly workout or are an athlete in training, then you really must add the above recipe to your own breakfast menu.

Ingredients:
½ a Cup of chopped & frozen Banana
1 handful spinach (small)
¼ ripe & pitted avocado
1 handful frozen berries
1-½ teaspoons of hemp seeds (shelled)
1 tbsp. cacao nibs (raw)
¼ tsp. powdered wheatgrass
¼ chopped cucumber
1 cup of coconut oil water

Process: Make sure the bananas have been frozen and are solid before placing all ingredients into the blender. Mix them all until the texture is smooth. If the texture becomes too thick, add a bit of water. Drink early in the morning.

Recipe 3: Peach Milkshakes

Milkshakes are very popular and known for providing good nutritional value in the mornings. They taste great and are good with any fruit you decide to use. According to latest research if you add two tablespoons of coconut oil then it is ideal. Coconut oil is known for having so many health benefits and also increases metabolism generally.

Ingredients:

1 Cup of almond milk or perhaps hemp seed milk
1 Cup of fresh/frozen peaches
½ Cup of fresh Pineapple Juice
½ Cup of frozen banana
1 tsp. of Coconut Oil

Process: Using a clean and dry blender, place all the above ingredients in and blend well. Keep going until it makes a smooth, fine milkshake. You can have this on its own or with a small meal.

Recipe 4: Quinoa Pancakes

Quinoa is considered a "superfood" because of its high protein, iron and fiber content. This makes it perfect for vegetarians. It has a very delicious nutty and grainy taste. Plus, it's also gluten free.

Making a proper, healthy breakfast will require some effort. Below we have the recipe for quinoa pancakes. They're full of protein, gluten-free, and a great start to any day. These can be made for lunch as well. Make sure you soak the quinoa overnight. This recipe will provide you with a very healthy meal and it will be very tasty too!

Ingredients:
½ a Cup of Quinoa
½ a Cup of water
A little Coconut Oil
1 tsp. of salt
Maple Syrup (topping)

Process:
- Place quinoa into the bowl and add four cups of water. Soak it at least eight hours. Soak Quinoa overnight. When it's ready, drain it then rinse it. Place the quinoa and some salt (1 teaspoon) into the blender.
- Add a ½ cup of water then grind. Ensure the batter isn't too thin or too thick. It should have a moderate consistency. If it happens to be a little too thick just add some water. If it turns out too thin just add some quinoa.

- Heat coconut oil in a pan over a medium heat. Add a ¼ cup batter into the oil once it's heated a little then cook for about 1-2 minutes until bubbles start to appear and corners become a golden brown color.
- Turn the pancake over and cook another minute. Ensure both sides are properly cooked. Remove it from the pan and serve it with some fruit topping, maple syrup, honey, or cream.

Recipe 5: Easy Cheesy Eggs

Ingredients:
¼ tsp. butter
1 tsp. whole milk
1 egg
1 tbsp. chopped tomato
1 tsp. grated parmesan
1 tsp. chopped chives
Muffins

Process:
- Add 1 tsp. of whole milk into a pan with 1 tsp. of parmesan and a ¼ tsp. butter. You will boil this for around 2 minutes until bubbles appear.

- Now add an egg to the pan along with the chopped tomato on the top. Broil for 7 minutes then set aside for about 2 minutes.
- Scatter 1 tsp. chives if you like and serve it as is or with a muffin (whole grain).

Recipe 6: Huevos Rancheros Sandwich for Breakfast

Ingredients

1/3 of a cup refined beans

2 Muffins (toasted & halved)

2 eggs

Salt

Pepper

Salsa

1 ripple of Avocado

Process:

- Half and toast 2 muffins. Peel the avocado then mash it using a fork. Add some salt to the avocado. Heat the beans until they are warm. Spread bean mixture on the muffins. Place the avocado on the muffin top.
- Over a medium heat place a pan greased with some olive oil. Crack into it 2 eggs. Add a little salt and cook for about 1 - 2

minutes. Now flip the eggs onto the other side carefully. Season with a little salt and pepper once again.

- Once cooked, place the eggs onto the muffins, add the salsa and the avocado then serve.

Recipe 7: Healthy Spinach Omelet with Goat's Cheese

Ingredients:
1 egg
1 tsp. of Canola Oil
1 Cup Baby Spinach
1 tbsp. crumbled goat cheese
Process:

- In a frying pan (preferably non-stick), and on a medium flame, add 1 teaspoon canola oil.
- Add 1 egg to the frying pan and then spin it. Now cook for about a minute.
- In the same pan sauté the baby spinach for another minute.
- Pour the canola oil and the goat's cheese onto the egg.
- Garnish with some baby spinach then roll it and cut it into half. This is a great breakfast

to have on the menu list and is very
nutritional.
- This breakfast will provide you with 2
grams carbohydrates, 1 gram fiber, 17
grams fat, 301 mg sodium, and 198
calories.

Recipe 8: Poached Eggs Marinara

Ingredients:
½ Cup Marinara Sauce
¼ Yellow Onion
Olive Oil
Red pepper

Process:
- Heat 2 teaspoons of olive oil in a pan on a
medium flame. Add ¼ yellow onion and
sauté until brown. Now add a little red
pepper and ½ cup of the marinara sauce.
- Allow the sauce to heat for about a minute
then add an egg. Cover your pan and leave
it on a low heat for about 7 minutes.
- Serve the poached eggs with wheat pita
bread or with any bread of your choice.

Recipe 9: Scrambled Eggs Tex-Mex Style

Ingredients:
1/8 Jalapeno
2 eggs
Corn tortilla
¼ diced bell pepper (red)
1 tbsp. chopped cilantro
1 tbsp. good cheddar cheese
Tomato
1 Onion

Process:
- In a smallish skillet add 1 tsp. canola oil and allow it to heat.
- Add one corn tortilla then pan fry for two minutes on each side. Now remove tortilla from the heat. Dice it well.
- Using the same skillet, sauté the jalapeno, the red and green bell peppers, the onion and tomato.
- Whisk the 2 eggs. Add them along with the vegetables to the same pan. Stir it into the tortilla then add 1 teaspoon chopped cilantro and cheddar cheese.
- A breakfast like this is nutritious and healthy. It has only 308 calories, 17 grams fat, 4 grams fiber, 21 grams carbohydrates,

17 grams protein, and 203 milligrams of sodium.

Recipe 10: Creamy Breakfast Pudding (Vanilla)

Ingredients:
¼ tsp. good vanilla extract
1 egg
Rice cereal
1 tsp. of sugar
¼ tsp. cinnamon
2 tbsp. chopped peach

Process:
- Whisk 1 egg in a bowl.
- Prepare the rice cereal going by its package directions. Don't add salt but put it into the saucepan itself.
- Now whisk the egg and the cereal until it makes a mixture. Add the vanilla extract, ¼ tsp. cinnamon, and 1 tsp. of sugar. Simmer for about 2 minutes then add the chopped peach as the topping.

CHAPTER 4: LUNCH

Lunch Recipe 1: Greek Salad and Pita Croutons

Ingredients:
Tomatoes (your choice of how many)
Cucumber (chopped)
Red Bell pepper (sliced) *Optional
Feta cheese (reduced fat if you prefer)
Olives (your choice of how many – chopped or whole)
1 whole grain pita
1 juiced lemon
1 Tbsp. of olive oil
Salt & pepper

Process:
- Whisk the lemon juice, olive oil, salt, pepper in a small bowl.
- Toast whole grain pita until it is crunchy. Chop into pieces.
- Mix the other ingredients in a bigger bowl. Pour the lemon dressing over the top. Drop pita pieces on top.

Lunch Recipe 2: Zucchini & Rosemary Flatbread

Ingredients:
½ cup zucchini

1 whole grain flatbread

¼ cup of mozzarella

2 tbsp. sliced almonds

1 tsp. sliced rosemary

1 cup halved grapes

Process:

- Preheat oven to 350° F. Heat whole grain flatbread on a baking sheet about 7 minutes or until crispy.
- Remove baking tray from oven. Top with ½ a cup of sliced zucchini, ¼ cup partly skimmed grated mozzarella, 1 tsp. of dried rosemary and bake for about 7 minutes or until cheese has melted.
- Mix the grapes and almonds.
- Serve with grape salad.

Lunch Recipe 3: Thai Shrimp Po'Boy

Ingredients:

2 ounces shrimp

3 tbsp. chopped avocado

¼ cup shredded carrots

2 tbsp. chopped cilantro

1 tbsp. of lime juice

2 tsp. chili garlic sauce

¼ cup sliced cucumber

Process:

- Cook 2 ounces shrimp (remove tails first) in 2 tsps. chili garlic sauce.
- Cut the roll lengthwise. Fill with shrimp, avocado, cucumber, & carrots.
- Top with lime juice and cilantro then serve.

Lunch Recipe 4: Pasta Salad and Tuna
Ingredients:

3 ounces of tuna

1 ½ oz. whole grain pasta

½ cup halved grapes

Tomatoes

3 tbsp. pitted & sliced black olives

½ cup drained & quartered artichokes

2 tsp. olive oil

1 tbsp. lime juice (fresh)

Salt and pepper

Process:

- Cook pasta then drain and allow to cool.
- Mix the rest of the ingredients together with the pasta.
- Lastly, add salt & pepper before serving.

Lunch Recipe 5: Savory Soup in the Slow Cooker

Ingredients:
1 cubed sweet potato (large)
2 cups sliced carrots
1 cup of fresh or frozen green beans
½ cup chopped fresh cilantro
1 small diced onion
1 clove minced garlic
2 (15 ounce) cans of drained & rinsed black beans
½ tsp. red pepper (preferably crushed) flakes
1 tsp. of chili powder
½ tsp. black pepper
1 tsp. of cumin
Sea salt or Kosher
2 cups low sodium vegetable broth
2 cups of vegetable juice

Process:
- Place all the ingredients into a slow cooker then cover and allow to cook for 6 to 8 hours on low, or until the vegetables are tender. Add 1 tablespoon cheddar cheese to taste.
- Now sauté the onion in the olive oil about 5 minutes or until it becomes tender. Put the

garlic into the cooker with all the other ingredients on the list.

- If you choose to you could add about two cups of chopped up kale at the last minute.

Lunch Recipe 6: Bean & Spinach Burrito Wraps

Ingredients:

1 x15 ounce can of rinsed and drained black beans
6 cups loosely packed baby spinach
1 ½ cups cooked Mexican or brown rice
½ cup chopped romaine lettuce
½ cup grated cheddar cheese, (preferably reduced-fat)
6 tbsp. fat-free Greek yogurt
½ cup of Salsa
Sea salt (or Kosher) to taste
6 whole grain (8") tortillas or wraps

Process:

- Preheat the oven to 300°F and warm the tortillas.
- Chop up the spinach then heat it in a big skillet on a medium heat for about 3 minutes or so.
- Place even amounts of bean and spinach mixture into the middle of the wraps. Place ¼ cup rice on each wrap. Add salsa, lettuce,

cheese and the Greek yogurt all over the
wraps.
- Fold wraps and then serve.

Lunch Recipe 7: Vegetable and Quinoa Stir-Fry

Ingredients:
2 cups of vegetable broth (or chicken)
1 cup quinoa (pre-rinsed)
1 tablespoon olive oil and sesame oil
½ cup minced green onions
1 cup finely diced carrots
2 cloves minced garlic
½ cup thawed frozen peas
2 lightly beaten eggs
Sea salt (or Kosher) to taste
2 tbsp. of soy sauce

Process:
- Add the quinoa and your choice of broth
  into a saucepan and bring to a boil. After it
  boils, reduce heat and allow to simmer for
  about 15 minutes or until liquid is
  absorbed. Place it to one side to cool then
  refrigerate for about two hours before stir-
  frying.
- Heat large skillet on a medium flame. Add
  the green onion, carrots, and cover until

tender. Cook for about 8 minutes then add the garlic.

- Add the quinoa and the broth in medium saucepan. Turn onto a medium to high heat and cover. Allow it to come to the boil and then reduce heat and allow it to simmer. Cook it until the liquid is completely absorbed. This will take around 15 minutes or so.
- Remove from the heat and let it cool. Refrigerate the quinoa for about two hours. You can save some time if you cook the quinoa the day before. Add peas to the quinoa then cook for another six minutes.
- If you like you could add eggs. Should you decide to do this, push the quinoa to the skillet sides and scramble the eggs in it. Make sure the eggs are scrambled well then stirred well.
- Add soy sauce and then cook for another minute or so before serving. Enjoy.

CHAPTER 5: DINNER

Dinner Recipe 1: Arugula, Sunflower Seed and Grape Salad

Ingredients:
2 tbsp. toasted sunflower seed kernels
3 tbsp. of vinegar
2 tsp. of grapeseed oil
1 tsp. of maple syrup
1 tsp. of honey
½ tsp. mustard, stone ground
7 cups baby arugula
2 cups halved red grapes
1 tsp. fresh thyme, chopped
¼ tsp. ground black pepper
¼ tsp. salt

Process:
- In a small bowl combine the honey, vinegar, syrup then mustard. Add the oil gradually and whisk it in.

- In a larger bowl, place arugula, seeds, grapes, and the thyme. Drizzle the vinegar mixture all over the arugula. Now add salt, pepper and gently toss to coat.

Dinner Recipe 2: Poached Eggs and Vegetable Hash

Ingredients:
1 cup chopped Vidalia

4 tsps. olive oil (Virgin preferred)

1 cup red potatoes (small potatoes and ¼ thick)

1 cup diced zucchini

1 cup diced yellow squash

1 tsp. dried herbs

1 cup trimmed ½" cut green beans

½ tsp. black pepper (ground and divided)

½ tsp. sea or Kosher salt

2 cups chopped seeded tomato

2 tbsp. thinly sliced chives

2 tbsp. chopped parsley (flat leaf)

1 tbsp. vinegar (white)

4 large eggs

1 oz. (¼ cup) shredded Parmesan cheese

Process:
- In a large skillet (nonstick) add the oil. Heat over a medium to high heat. Add the onion, herbs, and potatoes. Spread the mixture making sure it's in one single layer. Cook for about 4 minutes, (don't stir), or until the potatoes become slightly browned.

- Reduce to medium heat and add the zucchini, beans, yellow squash, salt, and only a dash of pepper. Now cook for about 3 minutes then remove the pan from the heat and cover. Let it stand for about 5 minutes. Add the tomato, parsley and chives, and stir it all in.
- Add some water to skillet, about 2/3 level. Bring it to the boil and reduce heat. Add the vinegar and stir. Once it is well boiled, break the eggs into a small custard cup then gently pour them into the skillet. Cook until it's done – about three minutes.
- Divide mixture into 4 plates evenly by carefully removing eggs from pan. Top every plate with an egg serving then sprinkle some cheese and black pepper to taste.

Dinner Recipe 3: Sweet Potatoes Oven-fried

Ingredients:
4 peeled sweet potatoes (medium sized & cut into ¼ inch slices)
1 tablespoon olive oil
¼ tsp. of pepper
¼ teaspoon salt
1 tbsp. finely chopped fresh parsley

1 tsp. orange rind (grated)
1 small minced garlic clove
Vegetable oil cooking spray

Process:

- Combine the sweet potatoes, olive oil, salt and pepper in large bowl. Toss gently to ensure they are well coated.
- On a baking sheet (large one) assemble the sweet potatoes and bake them at 400°F for around 30 minutes. Turn potatoes to the other side and allow to bake for another 15 minutes or so.
- Take a big bowl and add the parsley, garlic, and orange rind. Stir well. Now sprinkle parsley mixture all over the sweet potatoes.

Dinner Recipe 4: Stuffed Mediterranean Style Chicken Breasts

One of the healthier ways of increasing protein levels is through eating chicken. When it's made with some feta cheese, red pepper, and some olives it's extra tasty too. This will help boost your energy and ensure that the sodium levels and calories you are eating are at appropriate levels. It is entirely up to you how to cook it. You might prefer to sauté the chicken with some quinoa or you could grill it.

Ingredients:
8 boneless, skinless chicken breasts (approx. 6 ounces)
¼ cup or 1 ounce of feta cheese (crumbled)
1 large red bell pepper
2 tbsp. finely chopped Kalamata olives (pitted)
1 tbsp. minced basil (fresh)

Process:
- Cut the bell pepper lengthwise. You must ensure the seeds are removed as they do not taste very good in a meal.
- Preheat the oven and put the peppers onto a baking tray.
- Broil the chicken until it becomes dark brown.
- Prepare the grill to a medium heat. Combine the cheese, olives, bell pepper, and the basil.
- Cut the chicken breast so that it makes a small pocket that you can stuff. Cut the chicken breast horizontally and from the middle. Make sure you don't halve it.
- Now fill the chicken pockets with the mixture of bell pepper and some salt and

pepper. Grill the chicken. You must grill both sides for around 6 minutes. Make sure both sides are done.

- Now remove from grill and cover loosely with some foil. Serve.

Dinner Recipe 5: Beef Tenderloin with Gremolata Crusted with Peppercorn

Ingredients:
4 beef tenderloin (approx. 1" thick and trimmed) steaks
Cooking spray
4 tsps. canola oil
½ tsp. salt
2 tsp. black pepper
¼ cup flat-leaf chopped parsley
3 tbsp. chopped cilantro (fresh)
1 ½ tsps. chopped garlic
1 tsp. fresh oregano (chopped)
½ teaspoon lemon rind (grated)
1 tbsp. of fresh lemon juice
¼ tsp. of crushed red pepper

Process:
- Heat the oven (medium heat)
- Coat the steaks with canola oil, ½ of the salt mixture, and some pepper. Add steaks

to the pan then cook for about 3 minutes on each side until they're done well (or to your liking).

- In a bowl combine the rest of the ingredients and add 1 tablespoon oil, the parsley, and the rest of the salt.

Dinner Recipe 6: Arctic Char Fish & Relish of Orange &Capers

Ingredients:
4 Arctic char fillets (6 ounces)
2 tbsp. red onion (slivered)
1 cup of orange sections
1 tsp. orange rind (grated)
1 tbsp. freshly squeezed orange juice
1 tbsp. fresh chopped parsley (flat-leaf)
1 tbsp. minced capers
1 tbsp. olive oil (extra-virgin)
1/8 tsp. red pepper (ground)
½ tsp. sea salt
½ tsp. black pepper (ground)
Cooking spray
1 tsp. of rice vinegar

Process:
- Combine the orange sections, orange juice, orange rind, red onion, parsley, capers,

olive oil, rice vinegar, and ground red pepper in a bowl. Toss them all until well combined.

- Heat a skillet over medium heat. You will probably need a large skillet for this.
- Sprinkle the fish with the salt and the pepper then place it in the pan.
- Cook fish for about 4 minutes either side or until it's cooked well.
- Place each fish onto a plate then top with about ¼ cup relish.

Dinner Recipe 7: Nectarine Salsa and Chicken Kebabs

Ingredients:
1 ½ pounds of boneless, skinless chicken breast cut into 24 pieces of 2-inches each
Cooking spray
1 tbsp. olive oil (virgin)
1 tbsp. brown sugar
1 tbsp. lime juice (fresh)
1 tsp. minced garlic (bottled is ok)
2 tsps. chili powder
½ teaspoon cumin (ground)
¼ tsp. fresh black pepper (ground)
½ tsp. sea salt
1 large chopped red onion (approx. 2" pieces)

½ cup diced red bell pepper
2 cups of diced nectarines
¼ cup thinly sliced red onion
1 ½ tbsps. lime juice (use a fresh lime)
2 tbsps. cilantro leaves (fresh)
2 tsp. jalapeño pepper (minced & seeded)
½ cup diced and peeled avocado
¼ tsp. salt

Process:

- Preheat the broiler then add the chicken breasts, garlic, lime juice, olive oil, chili powder, brown sugar, cumin, salt, and black pepper to a shallow dish. Allow it to stand for about 15 minutes or until you can handle the chicken without burning your fingers.

- Place chicken pieces and chopped onion onto the skewers. Place skewers on broiler pan. Coat them all very well with the oil.

- Combine the nectarines, cilantro, bell peppers, lime juice, jalapeno pepper, salt, and peeled avocado into a bowl. Stir gently. You might want to add some more salt to taste. It's up to you.

Dinner Recipe 8: Roast Chicken

Ingredients:
1 whole chicken for roasting
2 tsp. softened unsalted butter
1 ½ tsp. minced fresh thyme
1 tsp. of paprika
2 tsp. olive oil (extra-virgin)
1 tsp. coriander (ground)
¾ tsp. salt
2 minced garlic cloves
¼ tsp. black pepper (freshly ground)
3 peeled & halved shallots
1 quartered lemon
3 fresh sprigs of thyme

Process:
- Preheat oven to 350°F.
- Clean the chicken and remove any excess fat.
- In a smallish bowl combine the butter, thyme, paprika, coriander, olive oil and salt. Rub it well into the chicken.
- Place the well-marinated chicken onto a rack in a roasting pan. Now place the lemon and thyme sprigs into the chicken's cavity.

- Place chicken onto a baking tray. Bake at 350 degrees for about 45 minutes.
- When it's done remove and serve with a sauce of your choice or even some French fries.

CHAPTER 6: SALADS AND SNACKS

Salad & Snack Recipe 1: Skinny Peanut Butter Yogurt Dip

Almost all of us have some cravings every now and then. Sometimes we want something sweet. The recipe below will give you both the sweetness and the nutritional value; so don't be afraid to try this one.

Peanut butter happens to be very protein rich. It also contains dietary fiber. It's a great way to satisfy a hunger pang and also keep sugar levels under control. You can enjoy this sweet and nutritional dish at home anytime.

Ingredients:
¼ cup crunchy, natural peanut butter
½ cup fat-free Greek yogurt (plain)

Process:
- Combine all the above ingredients in a bowl and refrigerate for an hour or until it's ready to consume.
- Serve with fruit or vegetables of your choice.

Salad & Snack Recipe 2: Peanut Butter Banana Cups

Healthy and clean eating is also about controlling calories. This must be done in order to maintain a weight that is healthy. However, as mentioned above, sometimes all of us like to have something sweet. This is a great recipe for boosting sugar levels quickly.

This recipe combines bananas with some peanut butter and this provides taste as well as controlling calories. We have suggested dark chocolate be used due to its lower sugar content and many flavonoids. The peanut butter is for some protein and the banana is for antioxidant content.

Ingredients:

¼ cup natural peanut butter
¾ cup dark chocolate cut into smaller pieces or chocolate chips (just make sure it's dark chocolate)
1 tbsp. unrefined melted extra virgin coconut oil (you can use regular coconut oil if you cannot find the extra virgin)
1 medium banana peeled then sliced into 16 rounds
16 pieces of 1.25 inch-baking cups

Process:

- Melt the chocolate in a saucepan and double boiler on low heat.
- Add it to the peanut butter and coconut oil.
- Place baking cups on a sheet.
- Add a layer of melted chocolate on the bottom of every baking cup. Add banana slice and a teaspoon of the peanut butter mixture. Coat this with some more chocolate then freeze for about an hour.
- Add a tbsp. powdered sugar if peanut butter becomes soft too quickly, before adding to baking cups.

Salad & Snack Recipe 3: Cucumber & Watermelon Salad

There are times when we all feel hungry but we don't want anything heavy. We still need to satisfy that craving, however. This recipe is quick and easy and will give you the satisfaction you need and is great for the summer when you also need something to cool you down.

Ingredients:

Lime Vinaigrette
½ tbsp. olive oil (extra-virgin)
1 tbsp. lime juice (freshly squeezed)

2 tsp. raw honey

¼ tsps. black pepper

¼ tsp. Sea salt or Kosher

Salad

4 cups of bite-size cubes of seedless watermelon

1 rinsed cucumber (large) cut into small triangle pieces

½ cup crumbled feta cheese

12 mint leaves (fresh) sliced into ribbon pieces

3 whole mint leaves (for the garnish)

Process:

- Place the mint leaves in 2 piles then slice them thinly into ribbon thin pieces.
- Whisk all ingredients for the dressing together.
- Add the dressing and the salad ingredients to a serving bowl then gently toss and coat well.
- Garnish with some mint leaves or mint sprigs if you choose.

Snacks & Salads Recipe 4: Mexican Corn Delicious

Ingredients:

4 corn pieces

1/3 cup Greek yogurt

½ cup finely grated cotija or añejo Mexican cheese or finely grated fresh Parmesan cheese

1 lime (wedges)

1 tablespoon chili powder

¼ cup finely chopped cilantro

Process:

- Fill a pot with water and add the salt. Bring to the boil.
- Add the corn and boil them for about 15 minutes or until the corn is done.
- Place the corn on a broiler pan. Broil for 5 minutes.
- Place corn and Greek yogurt together in a dish and sprinkle some cheese, lemon, chili powder, and the cilantro on the top.
- Make your choice of dressing and enjoy your meal.

Snacks & Salads Recipe 5: Caprese Style Pasta Salad

There are only 6-ingredients in this pasta salad so it's very easy to make. It is great for satisfying any odd pangs of hunger. Don't go for the junk food or full-calorie meals. The clean option is always the best option and it is also good for your health. This is a popular dish due to the fact that it is so easy to prepare, it is very healthy and it is also light on the stomach. A salad is always refreshing at any time and this particular one is another that's great for the summer months. It will provide you and your family or friends with a refreshing meal.

Ingredients:
4 cups whole grain pasta (cooked)
1 fresh, diced mozzarella ball (approx. 8-ounces)
8 Roma or 12 cherry tomatoes cut in half
Roughly chopped basil leaves
¼ cup olive oil (extra-virgin)
Sea salt

Process:
- Boil the whole grain pasta then set aside and let it cool.
- Combine all the ingredients (including the pasta) in a large bowl.
- Toss well and it's ready to serve.

Snacks & Salads Recipe 6: Turkish Sausage Balls

These Turkish style sausage balls can be made for dinner or as a side dish. You can try this with a wide variety of recipes. You might like to have these with rice or spaghetti or any type of gravy you like. Cooking is about creativity and finding ways to play with the taste buds.

These Turkish meatballs are basically small protein packed doses of food which are essential to keeping the immune system strong and active.

Ingredients:
1 pound lean ground turkey
1 tsp. fennel seeds (ground)
1 tsp. oregano (dried)
½ tsp. red pepper flakes (crushed)
2 tbsp. olive oil
½ tsp. salt
¼ tsp. pepper

Process:
- Mix all the above ingredients into a big bowl, mash well together and shape into balls.
- Add some oil to a pan and put it on medium heat. In batches, place meatballs into the pan and cook until they are brown on the outside and well-cooked inside. This will take about 8 minutes.
- After the actual cooking process, place them one by one on tissue paper in a dish and allow the excess oil to drain. Cover them with some foil to keep them warm while the other batches are cooking.

- When all of the batches have been cooked, serve them with some rice or pasta and a sauce of your choice.

Snack & Salads Recipe 7: Chicken Salad sans Mayonnaise

Ingredients
1 pound bite-sized chicken breast pieces
¼ cup olive oil (extra-virgin)
3 tbsp. freshly squeezed lemon juice
¼ tsp. pepper (black)
¼ tsp. sea salt
1 cup halved cherry tomatoes
½ cup celery (diced)
1 tbsp. dill (freshly chopped preferably, or 1 teaspoon of dried dill)
¼ cup parsley (chopped)
6 large lettuce leaves

Process:
- In a large enough skillet, add the olive oil (I-2 tablespoons) then place it on a medium heat. Add the chicken to the skillet and sauté until it changes color to a golden brown.

- Take a bowl and add the lemon juice, the salt and pepper, and the rest of the olive oil.
- When the chicken is properly cooked, add to the bowl then toss in the tomatoes, parsley, the celery, and the dill.
- Garnish with some lettuce leaves then serve and enjoy.

CHAPTER 7: DESSERTS

Dessert Recipe 1: Banana Split Black Forest Style

Ingredients:
2 bananas (cut lengthwise)
2 cups ricotta cheese (non-fat)
16 halved walnuts
1 tsp. unsweetened cocoa powder
2 tsp. of cherry concentrate

Process:
- Spoon the ricotta into a dessert dish then place one banana half on either side of the ricotta cheese.
- Put walnut halves on top of bananas then dust with cocoa powder.
- Now sprinkle cherry concentrate over the top and then serve. The ingredients above make 2 servings. If you would like more just double or triple the recipe depending on how many you would like.
- The nutritional facts for this recipe are: 377 calories, 40g carbohydrate, 23g protein, 11grams of fat, and 3.5 grams of fiber.
-

Dessert Recipe 2: Greek Yogurt with Mint and Oranges

Ingredients:
6 tablespoons fat free Greek yogurt
1 ½ teaspoons of honey
1 large peeled, sliced orange (slice it crosswise)
4 thinly sliced mint leaves (use fresh mint)

Process:

- Mix the honey and the yogurt together then pour mixture over the orange slices. Spread the mint over the top.
- This very nutritional recipe is so easy to prepare and contains only 171 calories, 11 grams of protein, and 34 grams of carbohydrates.

Dessert Recipe 3: Sandwiches of Chocolate Ganache

Ingredients:
1 ½ ounce semisweet chocolate chip bag
2-9 oz. boxes of Nabisco Chocolate Wafers
2 cups thick cream

Process:

- In a pan place the chocolate chips and thick cream and heat on a medium flame.
- Then remove from the heat, put in the fridge and allow it to chill a little.
- Once you have made the chocolate cream take two of the wafers then fill with the chocolate cream. Add a few ganache tablespoons too.
- Some of you may prefer the wafers stiffer. If so, you can make this a little before your occasion. If you prefer the wafers to be softer, make this dessert one day beforehand. The wafers will absorb the thick cream and ensure the dish is softer and creamier.

Dessert Recipe 4: Chocolate & Oatmeal Cookies You Don't Have to Bake

Ingredients:
2 full cups of raw fast-cooking oats
2/3 cup of peanut butter
¼ cup of cocoa
1 (3 ½ ounce) can of flaked coconut
1 teaspoon vanilla extract
½ cup of milk
2 cups of sugar
¼ cup of butter (or perhaps margarine)

Process:

- Add the peanut butter, vanilla, oats, cocoa, and coconut in a big bowl and mix them all well. Set it aside.
- In a saucepan place the milk, butter, and sugar, and bring the mixture to a boil. Cook this for about a minute stirring constantly.
- Now add the oat mixture and then stir again making sure it is mixed well together.
- Place it on a baking sheet. Allow it to cool.
- When it is cool you can serve it.

Dessert Recipe 5: Rum Balls Royale

Ingredients:

2 cups wafer crumbs (chocolate)

2 cups of gingersnap crumbs

1 cup of flaked coconut

1 ½ cups of powdered sugar (sifted)

1 cup toasted, ground pecans

1/3 cup chopped, pitted dates

1/3 cup rum (dark)

3 tablespoons corn syrup (light)

2 tbsp. melted butter (margarine will suffice if you don't have butter)

1 tsp. of vanilla extract

Some powdered sugar

Process:

- Place the gingersnap crumbs, the crumbed chocolate wafers, powdered sugar, coconut, pecans into food processor and blend everything together well.
- Add the rum, the corn syrup, and the butter and again make sure the mixture is blended well and binds.
- Take the mixture out of the food processor and shape it into small (but not too small) balls in the sugar or the gingersnap crumbs. Continue this process until all the mixture is finished.
- Refrigerate the balls to make them stiff and the binding stronger. Serve when ready.

Dessert Recipe 6: Rocky Road Brownies

Ingredients:

3 ounces chopped, unsweetened chocolate

½ cup or ¼ pound of butter

1 and 1/3 cup of sugar

1 tsp. of vanilla

2 eggs (large)

½ cup of flour (all-purpose)

1 cup marshmallows (miniature)

½ cup chopped walnuts

Process:

- Heat a pan over a low flame.
- Add the butter and the chocolate stirring them together until the mixture melts well.
- Take it off the heat then add the sugar, eggs, vanilla, flour, and the marshmallows. Make sure it is well blended.
- In an appropriately sized baking pan you must spread batter then sprinkle the walnuts over the top. Now bake batter at 350 degrees for about 30 minutes.
- If you want to check if it's done, use a dry, clean fork and insert it into the brownie. If it comes out dry it is ready to take out. If there is still some residue of the mixture on the fork then it needs a little more time in the oven.
- Remove it from oven and let it cool.
- When it has cooled sufficiently, cut into pieces (you can choose how big or small you want the pieces).
- You can also refrigerate them if you prefer a chilled dessert but ensure they brownies are covered if you plan on putting them in the fridge.

Dessert Recipe 7: Sugar Cookies (5 Ingredients)

Ingredients:
½ cup softened butter
1 ½ tsp. vanilla extract
3 cups divided powdered sugar
1 egg (large)
1 ½ cups flour (all-purpose)
Parchment paper
Nonpareils (white)

Process:
- Using an electrical beater and bowl, place the sugar and butter and beat at medium speed.
- Add the egg and the vanilla. Beat for another 30 seconds.
- Add the flour and then beat again ensuring it is all well combined.
- Make a dough and then place it on parchment paper. Flatten dough and using differently shaped cookie cutters, cut it into various shapes.
- Preheat oven to 375°F.
- Now grease a baking tray using flour then place cookies onto it and place in oven.

- Bake your cookies for about 10 minutes in batches until they have a lovely golden color about them.
- Once done, take them out of the oven. Set them aside and allow them to cool. This should take about 30 minutes.
- Finally, make a water/sugar mixture by placing sugar in a cup of water. Dip the cookies into the glaze and sprinkle them with nonpareils.
- Set them aside for about an hour.

Dessert Recipe 8: Blueberry Covered Frozen Yogurt

Ingredients:
40 drops of Stevia Extract
½ cup Greek Yogurt (plain and non-fat)
1/3 cup fresh, rinsed blueberries (dry them well)

Process:
- Add the yogurt, honey, and stevia in a smaller bowl.
- Add the yogurt then stir either the stevia or the honey, depending on your particular choice.
- Taking the blueberries, insert toothpicks into them then dip them into the yogurt

and push them with another toothpick. Repeat this procedure for the rest of the berries then put the pan in the freezer for about two hours.

- If you want to store blueberries you can place them in a sandwich bag before freezing.

Dessert Recipe 9: Delicious Strawberry Cheesecake

Ingredients:
½ a cup of fat-free cream cheese
½ cup of Greek yogurt (low-fat)
2 tbsp. of Coconut Palm Sugar
2 tsp. freshly squeezed lemon juice
¼ cup strawberries
4 dates
1/3 cup almonds (whole)
8 Dessert Dishes (mini), 3 or 4 ounces

Process:
- In a bowl, place the sugar, yogurt, cream cheese, and the lemon juice together. Make it into a very fine texture using an electric beater. You will have to beat this mixture around 3 minutes then refrigerate.
- Place strawberries in a bowl.

- Add the almonds to a food processor. Chop them then add the dates and allow it to pulse. Do not make this mixture too fine as it won't work well for this recipe.
- Divide mixture evenly into the dessert dishes and top them each with ½ a cheesecake and some yogurt batter.
- Now add strawberry mixture to the bowls and refrigerate for a minimum of 3 hours.
- You will achieve a better result with this dessert if it is made ahead of time, placed in the fridge and taken out just before serving.

Dessert Recipe 10: Non-Baking Coconut Snowballs

Ingredients:
2 tsp. melted coconut oil
1 ¾ cup shredded coconut (unsweetened & divided)
2 tbsp. unsweetened coconut milk
3 tbsp. good quality maple syrup
1/8 tsp. of sea salt
½ tsp. extract of vanilla
½ tsp. cinnamon (ground)

Process:
- Place only 1 cup shredded coconut and the coconut oil into a food processor. Process

on high speed. Continue mixing until the texture you have is fine. This texture should resemble a paste-like softness but no less. Make sure you don't blend it so well that it becomes as smooth as butter. This will not work well.

- In a big enough bowl add the coconut milk, the vanilla, cinnamon, salt, and maple syrup. Process until it is well enough combined. To this mixture you add the pulsed mixture, 2 tbsp. of shredded coconut. Now pulse again and combine them all well.
- Once the mixture is done well, shape it into balls then coat them with remaining shredded coconut.
- Refrigerate for an hour at the least before serving.
- You can keep these sweet delicious balls for up to 5 days in the fridge.
- Before eating take the balls out of the fridge and allow them to settle at room temperature. Enjoy!

CONCLUSION

Healthy and clean eating isn't something to be considered a luxury, nor is it to be considered a trend. It is an absolute necessity that every one of us will benefit from. Clean eating will result in a healthier lifestyle and therefore a healthier body.

In today's world with so many processed foods, we must make some very careful choices about what we put into our mouths and bodies. Artificially processed foods contain very high doses of sodium, unnecessary fats, and calories. None of these things are any good for our bodies.

At first, changing your eating habits may seem like a big challenge or even a burden. I can assure you, in the long run, this won't be the case. So many degenerative diseases could be avoided later on if we eat healthier now.

Many people in today's first world nations are prone to illnesses such as heart disease, kidney and/or liver failure, and definitely low immunity levels. So much of this can be attributed to unhealthy eating habits and lifestyles. We have ceased to make any effort in making and eating cleaner and healthier food due to our high stress, and time-limited lives. Processed food often taste good on the tongue due to the high levels of spices, or in most cases, the strong but artificial flavors, but these food items have a drastic impact on our bodies.

Healthy diets are those that are rich in healthy fats (remember that not all fats are bad – some are absolutely necessary), appropriate levels of carbohydrates, lean proteins, and a higher intake of water. Eating clean isn't just a diet. It is a lifestyle choice and it may take some time for the changes to really settle in with you, but you will be really thankful that you gave this gift to yourself. It is something worth trying.

Through clean eating your body and your mood will be much better. Simple meals with a combination of fresh fruits and vegetables are easy to make and so much healthier than artificial and processed food.

Apart from the health benefits of fruit and vegetables, the other great thing about them is they don't make your body acidic or feel too full and heavy which can lead to gastric issues, heart disease, and liver/kidney troubles. A healthy food change will result in better cell growth, the benefits of which you will see in your skin, hair, nails, and weight. Fresh fruit and vegetables are natural healers and have a bigger and better impact on health than any artificially processed foods.

We mentioned that clean eating is a good way to also maintain a good weight. Natural food doesn't make you put on weight or make the belly bigger and hang over your clothes. Fiber found in vegetables, for example, will actually help you naturally lose weight and the good news is they don't come with any side effects at all.

According to research, healthier, cleaner eating will result in building a stronger immune system. If your immune system is strong your physical and emotional body can handle a lot more. The research also suggests that clean eating can help cure certain illnesses faster and better than some unnatural medications.

Fruits, for example, can help kill harmful bacteria that may be lurking in the body. Think about this. If you love eating bananas, juicy mangoes, Vitamin C rich kiwi fruits, refreshing watermelon, you will be providing your body with some loving care and your body will respond in kind by being stronger and healthier for you.

This book is intended to encapsulate the main details of acquiring healthy eating habits and provides you with some recipe ideas to help you along the way. We also hope it has inspired you and given you the tools you need to begin making some changes that will last and have a positive impact on you and your family.

The recipes in this book are intended to accommodate a wide variety of tastes and preferences so you never get bored. We understand that some of you prefer heavier type meals and others prefer them light. We have tried to incorporate both of these meal types in this book all the while keeping in mind the basis of our intention – healthy, clean eating.

Please don't start wondering if you will ruin your budget if you start eating healthier and cleaner because in fact, the opposite is true. Try to think more broadly and carefully evaluate all the benefits of healthy eating while also calculating all the drawbacks of eating artificial or processed food. Don't risk the health of your family or yourself all for the sake of what will literally be only a few dollars. Invest in yourself and your health. Look after your body for it is the only one you have. Clean eating also provides benefits to your nervous system and will help you to sleep better.

When the immune system is strong and balanced, sleep becomes easier, the heart beats stronger, diseases and harmful toxins are slowly being eliminated from the body without the use of medicine. The skin doesn't age as quickly, hair is thicker and more beautiful, and there are no bloating or gastric problems too. What else can we really ask for?

Start today and use the instructions in this book to transform the artificial lifestyle you have to one of better health, better moods, and a more energetic body. Remain healthier for longer, sleep better and lead a potentially longer life with energy and joy.

THANKS FOR READING

We really hope you enjoyed this book. If you found this material helpful feel free to share it with friends. You can also help others find it by leaving a review where you purchased the book. Your feedback will help us continue to write books you love.

The Smart Reads library is growing by the day! Make sure and check out the other wonderful books in our catalog. We would love to hear which books are your favorite.

Visit:
www.smartreads.co/freebooks
to receive Smart Reads books for FREE

Check us out on Instagram:
www.instagram.com/smart_readers
@smart_readers

Don't forget your 2 FREE audiobooks.
Use this link www.audibletrial.com/Travis to claim
your 2 FREE Books.

SMART READS ORIGINS

Smart Reads was born out of the desire to find the best information fast without having to wade through the sheer volume of fluff available online. Smart Reads combs through massive amounts of knowledge compiles the best into quick to read books on a variety of subjects.

We consider ourselves Smart Readers, not dummies. We know reading is smart. We're self taught. We like to learn a TON about a WIDE variety of topics. We have developed a love for books and we find intelligence attractive.

We found that each new topic we tried to learn about started with the challenge of finding the pieces of the puzzle that mattered most. It can becomes treasure hunt rather than an education.

Smart Reads wants to find the best of the best information for you. To condense it into a package that you can consume in an hour or less. So you can read more books about more topics in less time.

OUR MISSION

Smart Reads aims to accelerate the availability of useful information and will publish a high quality book on every major topic on amazon.

Smart Reads hopes to remove barriers to sharing by taking the copyright off everything we publish and donating it to the public domain. We hope other publishers and authors will follow our example.

Our goal is to donate $1,000,000 or more by 2020 to build over 2,000 schools by giving 5% of our net profit to Pencils of Promise.

We want to Restore forests around the globe by planting a tree for every 10 physical books we sell and hope to plant over 100,000 trees by 2020.

Doesn't it feel good knowing that by educating yourself you are helping the world be a better place!? We think so too...

Thanks for helping us help the world. You Smart Reader you...

Travis and the Smart Reads Team

WHY I STARTED SMART READS

Every time I wanted to learn about something new I'd have to buy 20 books on the topic and spend way too long sorting through them and reading them all until I arrived at the big picture. Until I had enough perspectives to know who was just guessing, who was uninformed and who had stumbled upon something remarkable.

I wished someone else could just go in and figure that out for me and tell me what matters. That's how smart reads was born. I want smart reads to be a company that does all that research up front. Sorts through all the content that is available on each topic and pulls out the most up to date complete understanding, then have people smarter than me package the best wisdom in an easy to understand way in the least amount of words possible.

For example, I got a new puppy so I wanted to learn about dog training. I bought 14 different books about dog training and by the time I got through the first 5 and finally started getting the big picture on the best way to train my puppy she had grown up into a dog.

Yeah she's well behaved. She doesn't poop in the house. I can get her to sit and come when I call. But what if someone else went in and read all those books for me, found the underlying themes and picked out the best information that would give me the big picture and get me right to the point. And I'd only have to read one book instead of 15.

That would be amazing. I would save time. And maybe my dog would be rolling over, cleaning up after my kids and doing the dishes by now.That my friend, is the reason I started smart reads. Because I wanted a company I can trust to deliver me the best information in an easy to understand way that I can digest in under an hour. Because dog training is one of many subjects I want to master.

The quicker I can learn a wide variety of topics the sooner that information can begin playing a role in shaping my future. And none of us knows how long that future will be. So why not do everything we can to make the best of it and consume a ton of knowledge. And I figured all the better if I can also make a positive difference in the world.

That's why we're also building schools, planting trees and challenging ideas about copyright's place in today's world. Because as a company we have to be doing everything we can to support the ecosystem that gives us all these beautiful places to read our books. Thanks for reading.

Travis

Customers Who Bought This Book Also Bought

Probiotic Dieting: The Miracle of Probiotics in Healing Your Gut, Trimming Belly Fat and Weight Loss

Natural Ways of Boosting Testosterone: How to Bulk Up and Put Your Sex Drive in Overdrive

Mint As Medicine: Discover The Powerful Healing Properties of Herb in Treating Headaches, Allergies, Asthma, Clarity and Peace of Mind

The Powerful Benefits of Myrrh: Effective Myrrh Recipes For Healthy & Beauty, Oil Pulling Therapy, Creativity, Aromatherapy and Improving The Mind

Develop Self-Discipline: Daily Habit to Make Self Confidence and Will Power Automatic

How To Control Alcoholism: Proven Techniques to Stop Alcohol Abuse, Overcome Dependency, Break Addiction and Recover Your Life

How To Run: Beginner Running Program. Learn to Run. Running to Lose Weight. Runner Form. Fun Run.